KNOW YOUR OPTIONS:

THE DEFINITIVE GUIDE TO CHOOSING THE BEST DENTAL TREATMENTS FOR FAILING OR MISSING TEETH

Published by CelebrityPress®, Orlando, FL.

CelebrityPress® is a registered trademark.

Printed in the United States of America.

ISBN: 978-0-9983690-1-3
LCCN: 2016962894

Most CelebrityPress® titles are available at special quantity discounts for bulk purchases for sales promotions, premiums, fundraising, and educational use. Special versions or book excerpts can also be created to fit specific needs.

For more information, please write:
CelebrityPress®
520 N. Orlando Ave, #2
Winter Park, FL 32789
or call 1.877.261.4930

Visit us online at: www.CelebrityPressPublishing.com

KNOW YOUR OPTIONS:

THE DEFINITIVE GUIDE TO CHOOSING THE BEST DENTAL TREATMENTS FOR FAILING OR MISSING TEETH

By Dr. BRYCE GATES, D.D.S.

of Custom Dental of McKinney

CelebrityPress®
Winter Park, Florida

Good news!

Once a "top secret" solution for the rich and famous, today dental implants are available for almost everyone—and at a cost most people can afford.

CONTENTS

A COMMITMENT TO SERVE

Dr. Gates is very knowledgeable, trust worthy, and on top of the latest trends in the industry. He has helped myself and numerous friends & family with dental work and I highly recommend him.
~ Kurtis Kupfersmith

Not everyone has a great idea of what they want to be when they grow up, but I always knew that I wanted to be a surgeon. A vague term, in and of itself, but the concept of being a surgeon meant that I would be doing a service that helped other people in need.

By chance, I had an uncle and a cousin who were both dentists—a career that I never associated with the medical profession at the time—and I began to spend some more time with them. They took me over to their dental office and I was immediately drawn in, noticing a few things:

  ✓ The synergy in the office between the dentists and staff was exciting—everybody was happy to be there.
  ✓ The patients seemed relaxed and expressed gratitude for how they were being helped.

In general, it was a vibrant culture and I instantly loved it. But still… I wanted to be a surgeon.

Then on another visit, I played witness to something that I'd never thought of before—at least not in detail. My uncle was doing dental implants, and had started doing them over 30 years ago when it was still a very new and emerging technology. He was a pioneer. As I asked for more information, he shared insight that was quite compelling to me. He'd gotten started with implant dentistry so he could be of better service to the folks in rural Oklahoma, who were sometimes forced to drive a couple hundred miles for the types of dental treatments and services they needed.

My uncle's story inspired me, and as he shared more, I learned that there were often days where he did implants all day long. It taught me two things:

1. Peoples' problems with missing or failing teeth were more significant than I had realized, from an emotional perspective and from a health perspective.
2. Dentists can be surgeons, as well, if they choose to focus on specialty niches such as full mouth restoration, which is the umbrella that dental implants falls under.

From that moment on, I've never looked back. My interest has snowballed into a passion to serve others and restore their smiles.

After deciding on a direction in which I wanted to go, I spent the next decade focusing on doing what I had to in order to practice dentistry. It isn't easy to get into dental school so I committed myself to achieving academic excellence in high school, then undergraduate school, and eventually graduate school. I became a shadow behind every dental implant surgeon I could find, watching the procedures and observing the interactions between patients and dentists. I felt compassion for them, as well as understood the complete process—from emotional happiness to a healthier lifestyle—that encompassed implant dentistry.

I was working hard, but I didn't even realize how my honed in passion had really given me an edge, at first. An impactful event happened during my last year of dental school that highlighted just how much I'd learned. I was shadowing a periodontist when it occurred. At the time, these oral surgeons did most dental implants and as I watched, I saw these things they were doing that made me realize that all dentists who can do mouth restoration are not the same. Some of the differences were glaring to me and I wasn't sure how to respond. I admit, I wanted to interrupt and say something. Seeing how they'd lost sight of the patients' emotional needs, and even how they were physically feeling was so obvious to me. My keen eye and extensive experience watching these procedures allowed me insight into the moments when it was not going well—neither for the dentist nor the patient. These were professionals who'd been performing oral surgeries of some sort for a long time. I was just getting started, but I knew...

It was quite the conundrum, debating silence or saying something. It turned out that I didn't have to say anything at all, because the consensus quickly became that the procedure wasn't going to work for that day, and that they'd try again in a few months.

For me, knowing that I was going to focus on dental implants in my career, I determined that my training, education and know-how about all facets of the procedure would prevent situations like that from happening. With the proper pre-implant consultation and exam, it could have been avoided.

My exposure and repetition have made the difference in my life. This is not just with dentistry, but with everything.

The years are not everything, but how the experiences are evaluated and how many of them you have had are.

Today I am blessed to have a practice that offers the highest trained staff, best technologies, and a genuine love for our patients' wellbeing. And nothing will ever beat having a patient walk in to see me after a procedure with a sincere smile on their face and confidence from that smile showing in their every move.

Wonderful experience with everyone on the staff. Dr. Gates was awesome to work with, and I do mean work with. We discussed my current situation, went over my options for suggested treatments and answered my all of my questions. My treatments completed comfortably and beyond my satisfaction. No pain, lots of gain. Go see Dr. Gates and his awesome team. Be sure to ask about why he became a dentist. Great story!

~ Alton W

CHAPTER 1

THE PSYCHOLOGY OF MISSING AND FAILING TEETH

I am kind of embarrassed to say that I have let my teeth go over my adult life. I seem to do all the wrong things, such as drink sugary drinks, eat sugary food, haven't had regular dental care, etc. I am very unhappy with my smile at this point and time in my life. I was referred to Custom Dental by a Katy Davis and though it's a 2-hour drive to get there from my home I decided to give them a try. Such a great decision and well worth the drive. Dental care is expensive, there is no way around it. So, if you are going to pay for it anyway, why not go the extra mile to have the best work on my teeth? As soon as I walked into the office I felt welcome and as though I belonged there. The entire staff is fantastic! Very friendly and knowledgeable. If they don't know something they take the time out of their schedule to learn it. Dr. Gates is AMAZING, and makes sure his patients are as comfortable as possible. Thank you Custom Dental of McKinney for winning my business.

~ Jamie McCall

The Academy of General Dentistry (AGD) conducted a survey of dentists that was focused on better understanding the social impact of missing or failing teeth on peoples' emotional wellbeing. Out of the roughly 20,000 dentists surveyed, they found:

✓ 86% of their patients felt that tooth loss was a socially embarrassing problem

✓ 50% of patients who experienced tooth loss were less socially involved as a result

This was in comparison to patients who had a complete smile, an inviting smile.

The natural solutions to cope with this tooth loss were to consider full or partial dentures, dental bridges, or dental implants. The choice depended on the budget. The nuance—the satisfaction of the outcome, as well as overall mental health benefits—depends on the method of correction chosen.

In a world where we should be using our smile to change the world, we need to be mindful of how losing our smile can change us. I'm acutely aware of this every single day when I go to work and with every patient that I meet.

From the standpoint of one's psyche, missing and failing teeth can create significant impacts on the quality of life you experience, including:

✓ Job advancements and opportunities: a fear of talking and presenting your skills can happen with missing and failing teeth, often leading to you being overlooked for your dream jobs or opportunities for growth.

✓ Self-esteem and self-worth: when you fall into the mindset that you just want to blend in and not be noticed, it often happens, which leads to you feeling bad about yourself, despite being an amazing person inside that everyone would be honored to know better.

✓ Personal relationships: it can be challenging for individuals who lack confidence due to missing or failing teeth to establish positive, healthy relationships in their life. The embarrassment leads to more isolation than they desire, or than what promotes a healthier involvement in the world around them.

✓ <u>Your happiness level, in general</u>: when we are not happy, our quality of life goes down considerably and that is heartbreaking. We are wonderful beings meant to experience joy in our lives.

Our smiles are often our signature, and a genuine smile carries through into the way we carry ourselves and even the spark in our eyes. It means so much and it's a sign of friendliness, which is an important factor in opening up opportunities for greater happiness and fulfillment.

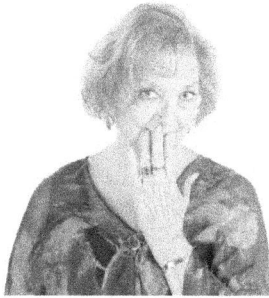

Imagine how wonderful it would be to go from covering up your beautiful smile to allowing others to see it without fear or embarrassment.

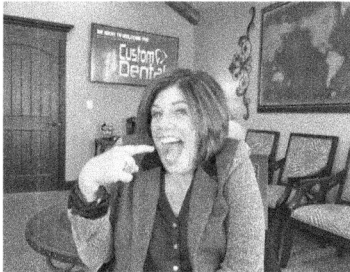

Aesthetically, we all have a desire to feel that we have acceptable appearances. A nice smile is one of the biggest of these aesthetic features that we look for in ourselves, and in those we meet. A nice, warm smile is hard to forget. But in addition to that, there are other concerns that stem from missing or failing teeth that impact us aesthetically, which does have an emotional impact. These things include:

✓ <u>Looking older than you actually are</u>: let's face it—no one wishes for this, but the facial structure does shift when there are missing teeth, often creating the illusion that you are older than what you are.

✓ <u>Causing the chin to recess</u>: a recessed chin becomes something that makes many people self-conscious during those special moments in their life where there may be photo opportunities, or even that unexpected glance in a mirror that catches one off guard.

These adjustments in our appearance can be so tough on us, really impacting how we evaluate our self-worth. We all deserve to feel wonderful and let the world see what's wonderful about us. It's that simple, and these powerful reasons are a few of the biggest deciding factors for people who choose to go with implant dentistry today over dentures or bridges.

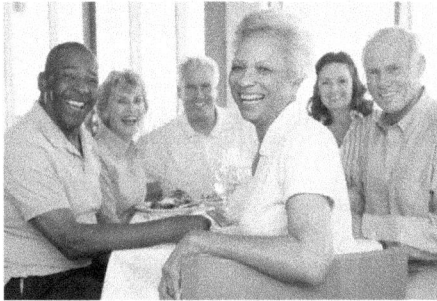

Another significant part of how we feel about ourselves stems from how we can interact and enjoy those social moments in our lives. A great example that many patients refer to involves what happens when they go out to eat. Most people with missing or failing teeth will do one of these things (and most likely all of them):

✓ <u>Not eat out of fear</u>: fear of spilling, drooling, and even losing a tooth by taking a bite of food exists. The thought of that being displayed is excruciating for some, so they choose to get clever and crafty by shifting their food around, claiming they're not as hungry as they thought, and then not enjoying a meal with everyone else. They only eat once they are in the privacy of their own home.

✓ <u>Not eat due to pain</u>: if it hurts when you take a bite of food it's hard to hide that. Just like if you accidentally get a bop to the nose, the pain can shoot up and reflect in your eyes as they gloss over or show your discomfort. It puts people in an awkward situation that they'd rather avoid.

✓ <u>Hesitant to laugh</u>: not unlike the fear to smile, people with missing and failing teeth are often hesitant to laugh. Furthermore, they create the habit that if they do by chance show their happiness, their hand automatically covers their mouth. Does this sound like something that you've been doing? If it is, you're not alone.

✓ <u>Changes in speech</u>: not all words sound the same when you have missing and failing teeth and that can make people feel quite self-conscious. Eventually, you grow quiet and don't participate in the conversation, which can leave you feeling isolated.

As you can see, the psychological impacts on missing and failing teeth are very challenging for those who are experiencing them. If you reflect on how this has possibly impacted your own life, or perhaps the life of someone you know and care about, you can see why there is every reason to restore that vibrant confidence and energetic smile that comes from knowing that your mouth is not a source of embarrassment. That's the power behind oral restoration.

If the personal motivating factors are not enough, the next chapter will cover the medical concerns that exist and are enhanced by missing and failing teeth. Teeth truly do impact all parts of our lives.

My experience at Dr. Bryce Gates today was great, his team and him made me feel really welcome and relaxed. I am going to recommend them to all my family and friends. They get 2 thumbs up from me.

~ Rosie S

CHAPTER 2

THE HEALTH CONSEQUENCES OF MISSING AND FAILING TEETH

Dr. Gates is so kind, gentle, and patient! He has an incredible heart and is passionate about helping people! He did extensive work on my best friend and walked her through fear unbelievably! He has completely transformed her smile, which has given her more confidence and better health! You won't regret choosing Dr. Gates @ Custom Dental in McKinney!

~ Tonia Amore

When you change your smile you don't just change your life for the better from an emotional capacity, but you are also taking care of promoting better health for you, which is important, as well.

Aside from oral health, there are possible consequences for other key areas of your health and body, including:

✓ Higher risk for heart conditions
✓ Depression
✓ Obesity
✓ Diabetes

✓ Joint inflammation
✓ Muscle and bone deterioration

All of these health challenges are significant and for the most part, once you have them they are irreversible. Thankfully, if their onset is due to missing or failing teeth, you have options to help manage them, which will increase your potential of having them not worsen. How important is this? To give you an idea: Mayo Clinic did research that showed that people who address oral health risks such as missing or failing teeth with permanent solutions, are likely to live 10 years longer than those who don't. We can all agree that there are a lot of smiles we can give and amazing experiences to have in a decade!

Take a few moments to think about the things we can do in order to be healthier. One thing is exercise, which is obviously good for us. The other main thing we can do is to be mindful of our diet, which means the foods we eat.

If you're suffering from failing and missing teeth, eating the healthiest foods you can suddenly becomes significantly harder. Fruits like apples become more challenging to eat, meats and other foods rich in protein are challenging, or even painful, to chew. We end up gravitating toward soft foods that may be high in fat and starches, low in nutrition, or is made from processed and preserved ingredients. You may be full, but you will also find that you are slowly depriving your entire body of the best type of nutrition to lead a healthier life. It raises an important question:

Isn't it a smarter choice, a brighter smile aside, to ensure you can eat foods that keep you healthier and provide you with more energy for a better day?

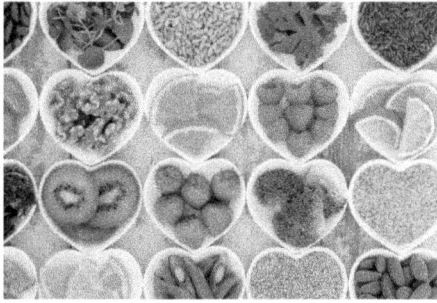

In addition, missing and failing teeth lead to deterioration of the jaw bone and atrophy of the muscles due to lack of use. Our mouths are designed to have teeth in them, both for structural support and for function. The main concerns that someone who has missing or failing teeth has if they don't take corrective action include:

✓ Periodontal disease (gum disease)
✓ Loss of bone mass—and once bone is gone, it is permanently gone
✓ Bad breath
✓ Temporomandibular Joint (TMJ) symptoms, which include: dizziness, Tinnitus (ringing of the ears), headaches, and soreness and stiffness in the neck, shoulders, and back

Even when we are at our healthiest, our mouths are at risk of deterioration if we don't use the proper oral hygiene. This means that we have to give the proper time and attention that our mouths deserve in order to counteract that deterioration. Furthermore, not addressing bacteria in the mouth gives it a chance to continue attacking more areas of the mouth, leading to further problems— yet, preventable problems.

A FEW FACTS TO CONSIDER

Bone loss is progressive…and cannot be reversed. Within 6 months of losing a tooth (or teeth) 40%-50% of your mouth's ridge bone is lost—permanently.

Our looks do change due to missing and failing teeth, including: looking older, facial collapse, and wrinkles around the mouth.

We experience nerve pain due to the raw, exposed nerves in certain areas with prolonged bone loss.

Dentures and partials only provide 40% to 50% of natural tooth function, at best.

The foods that are easiest to eat with missing and failing teeth are starchy and soft, which worsens the tooth condition, as well as overall health.

NOW THAT YOU KNOW

My sense of compassion for people who are embarrassed about their oral health problems, regardless of how they came to be, is strong. I understand how you feel and don't take that lightly. You do need to take a chance, though, and talk with a professional to build trust and gain the knowledge that they are going to do what's best for you. I meet with people every day who are involved in this journey of education and correction to some degree, whether it's a one-on-one consultation, someone attending a dental implant seminar I'm hosting, or they are preparing to start a corrective procedure with me.

It isn't a responsibility that is taken lightly, and it all begins with finding out what your exact condition is. You may have an idea, but without the right type of evaluation, you truly do not know the specifics to your case. Within those specifics are answers as to what the most effective treatment options possible are for you.

As a new patient, I was very pleased after my first appointment. The staff was very friendly and made me feel welcome. Dr. Gates took time to explain the procedure and pointed out a potential problem that I was not aware of from a previous dentist. He took special care to make sure I was comfortable during the procedure. Dr. Gates also took the time to personally call me the night before my appointment to welcome me to his office and even called me that night after my procedure to make sure I was ok and to see if I had any concerns or questions. I really appreciated that extra attention directly from the doctor after hours. From the attentive staff, to the beautiful office, to the modern state-of-the-art equipment I felt like I was in good hands and look forward to my next visit with Dr. Gates.

~ Mary C

CHAPTER 3

WHY DENTURES AND BRIDGES DO NOT WORK

For years I was afraid to go to the dentist, and my health and smile suffered. My friend suggested going to Custom Dental and for months I avoided going.... I wish I listened to her earlier!!! Dr. Gates and his team took the time to listen, answered my questions and made me feel so comfortable. This office knows how to make people feel welcome and like family! Thank you, Dr. Gates, and team!

~ Katy Davis

The two most common routes that people decide to take to address their missing and failing teeth are to either consider dentures or bridges. The main reason that these procedures are considered first is affordability. For a great many years they were considerably less expensive than dental implants. However, like all things in the market, the more commonplace it becomes, the more the price adjusts downward.

Today there is a lesser gap in the affordability of dental implants than one might think.

As you begin to evaluate all your options and solutions for mouth restoration, it is also important for you to note that dental implants are the only permanent solution, working successfully 98% of the time after ten years, which cannot be said for dentures or bridges. Furthermore, many of the people that are looking for a satisfactory solution to their missing or failing teeth have already tried dentures and bridges before they end up visiting our office. As a result, we help people who feel like they are on their last chance. But, with spreading the word and educating people as early as possible, we are hoping to shift this imbalance. It all begins with education.

THE BASICS OF DENTURES

Most patients first meet with me to ask about dentures, and this is okay. What I always like to share with them is a story to set their expectations about what dentures offer, exactly.

The best a denture will ever be is a wooden peg. Think back to the Civil War days—when a soldier lost a limb the best prosthetic they could offer was a wooden leg and some crutches. In this same era, if you had missing teeth, and you were lucky, you might get dentures.

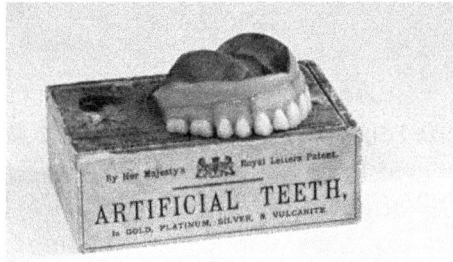

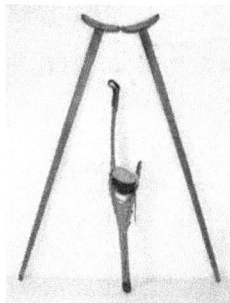

Fast forward to the present and take note of the differences. If you lose a limb there's no wooden peg option. You get a titanium articulated joint that will take the place of what's missing. This is also what a dental implant is—a premium replacement that is built for the long run.

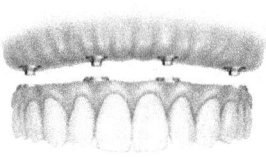
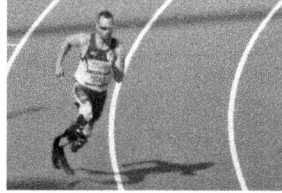

Dentures and bridges alike are a quick fix and an old-school solution for the aesthetic portion of mouth restoration. This is important, of course, because as already discussed, it relates to the emotional wellbeing of someone, which is imperative to their overall happiness. However, dentures come with their share of concerns as well. The most common complaints that people who've chosen dentures have include:

✓ They often slip, creating challenges for eating and talking, making it obvious that they have dentures.
✓ When you are eating certain foods you can experience pain when you bite down.
✓ The problems associated with the taste and ease of use of denture pastes and creams is awful—a minty flavor doesn't guarantee a fresh minty taste.

As a dentist, the complaints of our patients are certainly noted. The concerns we have from a professional side include what our patients are concerned about, but extend into things that we know from a medical professional's standpoint are also very problematic, including:

✓ Deteriorating bone quantity and density, which cannot be corrected.
✓ Atrophy of the muscles that are unused.

✓ Restriction of blood flow to the mouth, which can lead to further complications.

Before we begin, take a moment to do a little experiment to demonstrate the impact blood flow has on gum tissue, specifically how it can be impeded by dentures, causing accelerated bone deterioration.

Take your finger and press it into the back of your hand. Then lift it off after ten seconds. What do you see? You likely see a white, off color area in the shape of your pressed fingertip. Why is it there? It's there because you restricted the blood flow to those areas. That is exactly what happens with dentures and partials—they restrict blood flow, creating a risk of further trauma to the mouth at some point.

Most people know somebody who wears dentures, and if you spend a significant amount of time with them you've probably noticed that they often face a few challenges, whether it's the shifted speech patterns, a subtle clicking noise when they talk, or their overall inability to truly enjoy their food at meal time.

But how did they get to that point? What was their decision-making process?

As mentioned, money is a huge driving factor in choosing the types of dental procedures that you have done. It's understandable, of course, but the more you learn, the better able we are to show you why that little extra investment upfront with dental implants can save you a significant amount of money down the road, all while giving you a genuine, lifelong smile, not just a temporary fix.

When it comes to dentures, there are a few options out there that will be offered to people, depending on what their specific needs are. They include full dentures and partial dentures.

Full Dentures

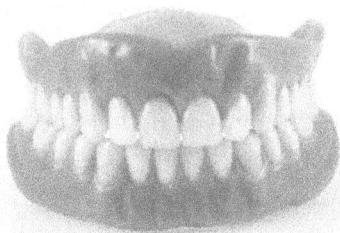

For complete tooth loss or seriously failing teeth, you have a choice of getting full dentures. There are options available: conventional and immediate. The main differences are:

✓ Conventional: this style of denture is ready for placement in the mouth about eight to twelve weeks after your teeth have been removed. The process of making it takes place after your remaining compromised teeth have been pulled; however, you spend up to three months without any teeth at all, which is not only uncomfortable, but potentially embarrassing and unhealthy for good nutrition.

✓ Immediate: with an immediate denture, it is made in advance of any tooth pulling procedures and positioned immediately afterward so you can wear it right away. This is advantageous over conventional dentures because you can wear teeth during your healing period. There are drawbacks, though, which include that your bone and gums will still shrink over time, particularly during the healing process. It's also highly uncomfortable, which makes it highly non-ideal. Plus, they are not as secure, which means that there are more adjustments, potential pressure spots, etc.

Regardless of the type of dentures that are used for a full denture option, you are going to continue to have reductions in bone density and atrophy of the unused muscles in the mouth. This means that there is no "one and done" option, standard dental visits aside. Every few years, at minimal, you'll likely need to address denture concerns, and possible replacement.

Partial Dentures

When people opt for partial dentures, they either have a single tooth that needs to be replaced or a series of teeth, but not the entire mouth. There are two types of partial dentures. They are differentiated by the strength and therefore longevity of their expected use. The more long-term partial denture has a custom casted metal framework that acts as a rigid support clasping around existing teeth supporting the false teeth. As demonstrated in the picture below. This is referred to as a partial denture.

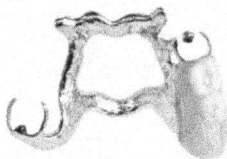

The partial denture also comes in a cheaper less stable form often referred to as an interim partial denture or "flipper". The difference between this partial and the one mentioned above is the absence of a metal framework. Because this partial is

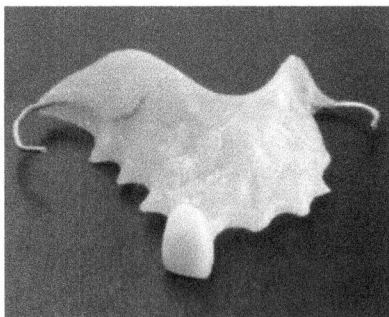

comprised of acrylic as its bulk it is much weaker and can break more easily and is therefore usually only intended as a temporary replacement after surgery while waiting on healing.

This is a popular option for most people because it is considered highly affordable and can be done in a relatively quick period of time. The drawbacks are quite substantial, though, and include:

- ✓ Damage to the natural teeth from force applied by the clasps, eventually leading to more tooth loss.
- ✓ There is a "gum colored" plastic plate that will be attached to it. This plate is most often uncomfortable, it's easy to get food trapped underneath it, and it's easier to have issues with poor breath because of it.
- ✓ Deterioration of muscle and bone continue.
- ✓ There is a high likelihood of having to replace a flipper denture every five to ten years.
- ✓ They have to be removed at night.

Overall, the maintenance remains high for these unnatural teeth.

There is an implant anchored denture partial available, which has benefits that include stopping bone loss and offer additional function; however, they still need to be removed at the end of the day and are not truly "permanent."

The next option that some people consider is a bridge.

Bridges

A bridge offers a more permanent solution, but it still does not address bone density loss and atrophy of the unused muscles in the mouth. Still, many people choose this option because it is more permanent. This is wonderful for aesthetics, but does nothing to address better health or full mouth function. Plus, it still has to be replaced every ten to fifteen years.

The more pressing fact on bridges is that they compromise adjacent teeth and if anything were to occur with those teeth in the future, it is no longer a one tooth problem, but a problem involving multiple teeth. This is because they are all fused together.

One of the most popular options for a bridge is the option called the Fixed Maryland Bridge.

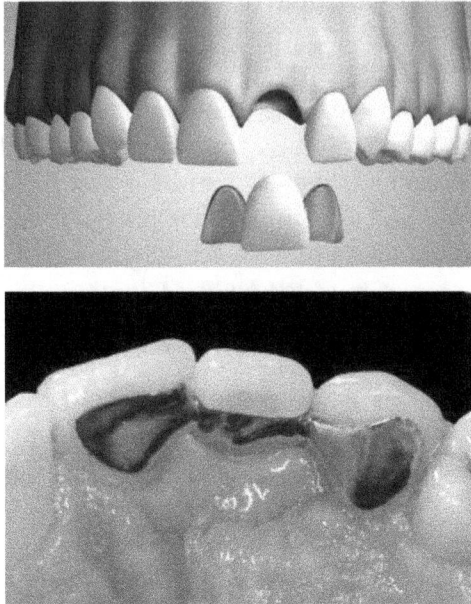

While it will work aesthetically, one of the most startling things about the Fixed Maryland Bridge is that you actually have to compromise two good teeth in order to have it placed. If you're suffering from missing and failing teeth that should be an alarming thought. Because the minute those healthy teeth become compromised they are susceptible to disease, bacteria, and going bad in the future.

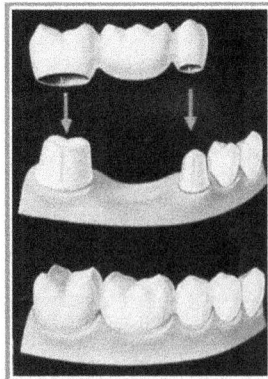

A step further for a bridge solution to tooth loss is the Fixed Bridge, which replaces one or more teeth by placing crowns on the teeth on either side of the space, and then attaching artificial teeth to them. This is what creates the bridge, and it is cemented into place. This solution does prevent other teeth from shifting; however, it still creates a vulnerability to your current teeth, and does nothing to address bone loss.

As a reminder, we keep mentioning bone loss, and this is highly significant because a loss of bone means a change in facial structure. As aesthetics and wanting to feel good about yourself are such driving factors, this is important to take note of.

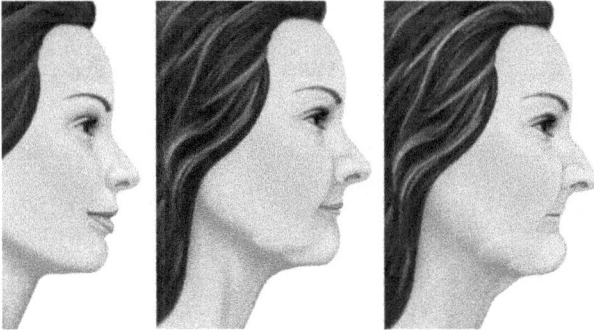

The Better Choice

One of the best things that come out of my consultations with patients, whether they currently have dentures or a bridge, or are considering it as a solution is that I can provide them the information they need in order to make a smarter decision. While monies are always a factor for patients—as they should be—there are also financial solutions that make it easier for a patient to look at dental implants as the smarter alternative.

When I first walked into the office in helping Custom Dental plan a Carter BloodCare blood drive I knew I had to change dental providers. The staff is amazing and they are very thorough and take time with you to ensure all your questions are answered. I felt important, not just another client through the door. My experience as a patient is more than outstanding and I will definitely be referring friends and family to Dr. Gates and his staff!

~ Sarah H

CHAPTER 4

THE BENEFITS OF DENTAL IMPLANTS

I found Dr. Gates and his staff to be extremely knowledgeable, most professional, and sensitive to my dental concerns. I felt immediately at ease as Dr. Gates and staff discussed my treatment options at length and laid out a plan, both dental and financial. The office environment is also warm, friendly, and inviting with the latest technology! No old-school stuff in this office! The staff really works very hard in assuring your level of comfort on each and every visit! Hey, I am pretty hard to please with high expectations and Dr. Gates with staff continues to meet and exceed those expectations every time! I urge anyone that is looking for a great dentist and staff, whatever your dental needs are to make an appointment with Dr. Gates. You will not be disappointed! But, you do not have to take my word for it. Give them a call, set up an appointment, and I promise you will not be disappointed as you have everything to gain!
~ Maurice Smith

Dental implants are a solution to long-lasting mouth restoration. With 98% of all dental implants being a success, they have proven to be well worth the consideration and cost by most every patient who has had them. Imagine the freedom that comes from:

✓ Being able to talk naturally, without concerns of a "lisp-like" sound or the clicking of dentures

✓ Smiling confidently
✓ Not having to have new dentures or bridges every five to ten years
✓ Eliminating unnecessary bone loss
✓ Stopping muscle atrophy in the mouth
✓ Not having to remove your temporary teeth nightly
✓ Reducing the risks of bad breath associated with dentures

All of this can take place by considering dental implants as your permanent solution to missing or failing teeth. Whether you have a single tooth that needs replacement, a few, or are in the rare situation to where all your teeth need to be replaced, you achieve great results for your life, which allow you to:

✓ Eat healthier
✓ Smile more
✓ Worry less
✓ Rebuild confidence

Does everyone qualify for dental implants? No, they do not. If any of these factors apply to you, you are not a candidate for dental implants:

✓ You are pregnant
✓ You are HIV positive
✓ You have uncontrolled diabetes

There may be other factors that would disqualify you from being a good candidate, but they are rare and considerably uncommon compared to the three mentioned above.

As we've shared (with great excitement), 98% of dental implants are a success. With a good oral hygiene routine and regularly visiting the dentist, you are likely to be good to go—for life. The 2% that fail are most often due to keeping poor oral hygiene habits or certain lifestyle choices that are bad for the body. For example: out of the 2% of fails, a majority of them are smokers.

This is important to consider and something that we certainly cover with all our patients who are exploring dental implants.

Other noted reasons for failures include:

✓ Contamination
✓ Infection
✓ Too much pressure during placement
✓ Excessive movement during healing
✓ 5%-10% of that 2% failure rate is from unknown causes

Are you ready to get serious about addressing the long overdue problem of your missing and failing teeth? Does the process of mouth restoration seem like a distant dream, one that you can't quite grasp? It's time to begin thinking about how you want your life to play out, and what you want the quality of it to be.

A BRIEF HISTORY OF DENTAL IMPLANTS

Dental implants are not a modern invention, although after I share their history with you, you are sure to be grateful for the modern approach.

Documentation of dental implants goes back to the Ancient Egyptian days, where they used little rocks, shells, and gold as dental implants. That was 3000 years ago!

After that, the technology did go to the side somewhat, as people chose to focus on dentures and partials, instead of permanent solutions. It was in the early 1980s when dental implants started gaining popularity again. New methods and techniques to help improve smiles and lives—new at the time and exciting. Yet, they are nothing like what exists today and what I can offer patients in my practice.

All of this is so exciting because it builds the story and research behind why we can transform smiles and therefore, lives.

THREE THINGS TO CELEBRATE WITH DENTAL IMPLANTS

Dental implants offer a solution when you are sick of losing quality of life and are ready to embrace everything you have to gain by having all your teeth and your smile back.

1. <u>Enhanced quality of life</u>
   There are many wonderful things that happen when we are confident in our smile and know that our mouth is in good condition both health-wise and aesthetically. Imagine gaining the confidence to apply for that new job. Be the happy, energized face in pictures, not the one who looks serious or mad, and is afraid to show their teeth. It's also easier to talk and communicate with others with ease, knowing that your teeth are in good condition and you don't have to be self-conscious about having "all eyes on you."

2. <u>That you had the confidence to act</u>
   When it comes to taking control of your health to live your best life, nothing is better than showing the initiative to take action and find out what your options are, exactly. No one can do this aside from a qualified dental implant practitioner. Every case is as unique as the individual, and you'll already begin to feel better just by taking action to meet with a specialist to find out all the information you need to know. This book has given you a great start, but it is an overview.

3. <u>Experience benefits that are guaranteed to make you smile</u>
   Life should not just be work and worry, it should also be an opportunity to celebrate special moments with people we love, explore, and feel wonderful while doing all those things. Dental implants allow you to talk more naturally, eat healthier foods, have a confident smile, make your facial structure more natural, and eliminate the worries that come from dentures and bridges.

WHAT DENTAL IMPLANTS DO FOR YOU

In the most basic sense, a dental implant is a permanent solution to addressing missing and failing teeth. Through evaluation and a plan of action, dental implants are used to replace teeth by mimicking nature in form and function, while restoring hope and a sense of optimism to the patient.

Because of their natural look and feel, dental implants offer a huge benefit to those who choose them because they are effortless to maintain and require only a minimal amount of healing time.

Most people return to work within one day of receiving dental implants, requiring only a dose of over-the-counter pain relief medicine to feel comfortable.

Creating comfort for patients who get dental implants is definitely a huge concern, both as a compassionate human being and a professional. The benefits extend beyond that, alone. Dental implants also are independent "structures," which means they don't require any surrounding teeth to be compromised or carry the load of the implant. Less stress on the mouth means better results with lesser risk of complications.

THE THREE PARTS OF A DENTAL IMPLANT

As in all areas of health and treatments, with time comes better knowledge on how to best solve medical problems. The same is true of dental implants. Where they were when they first began to where they are today being substantially different. The success rate alone is a stand-apart, impressive number; however, the way the dental implants are made that we use at our Custom Dental practice is truly revolutionary and done with state-of-the-art technology.

There are three basic parts to a dental implant: the titanium implant, the abutment, and the crown.

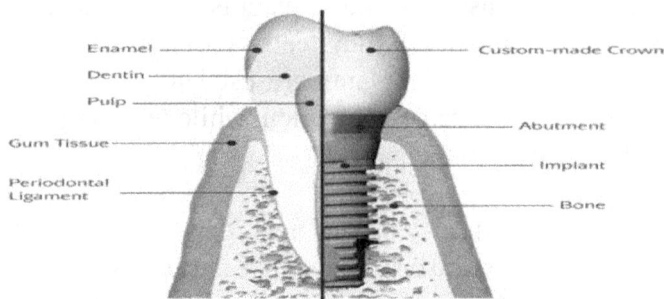

Enamel	Custom-made Crown
Dentin	Abutment
Pulp	Implant
Gum Tissue	Bone
Periodontal Ligament	

Let's go into what each of these parts does for the dental implant, exactly, and why the three parts as a whole become a dynamic, effective solution for restoring your smile and your health.

- ✓ The titanium implant: this is fused directly to the jaw bone. The reason that titanium is used over all other metals is that both muscle and bone respond to it, adapting to it and keeping their integrity as a result. This means no bone loss from missing teeth and no atrophy from unused muscles in that area. The process of the bone accepting the implant is known as osseointegration.
- ✓ The abutment: this is the portion of the dental implant that is secured over the titanium implant. It protrudes from the gum line, creating the base for the crown.
- ✓ The crown: this component is what looks and acts like a natural tooth. Made of zirconia, porcelain, or a high noble metal substructure, it is hard and sturdy and can perform any function that a natural tooth can, and in some cases even better. It's very sturdy and nearly impossible to break.

These three components, when put together and properly placed in the mouth, create a change for people who receive them that is so wonderful. The joy they experience is part of what keeps me so excited to keep promoting dental implants, performing the procedures on people every day, and seeing them during follow-up visits—a bright and grateful smile on their face.

To give you an idea of how the dental implant looks compared to the natural tooth, take a look at this side by side comparison, in which there are four implant teeth among the natural teeth:

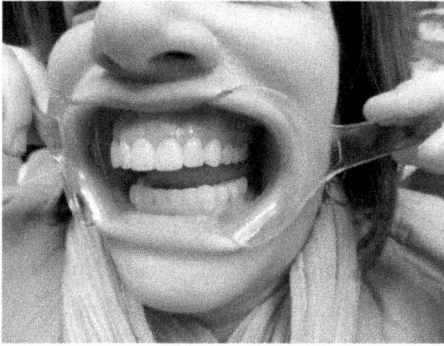

Think about how sensitive your mouth is to pain and discomfort, and how flair-ups can occur at any time, without warning, when you are dealing with missing and failing teeth. Then there are those who are always in pain and discomfort, which is very debilitating to a productive, happy life. Chronic, continuous pain takes its toll on everyone—emotionally and physically. Dental implants help to alleviate all of these things, making those tough times turn into distant memories.

THE HYBRID BRIDGE OPTION

This is a favorable option for many people who are looking to have an effective, permanent solution for missing or failing teeth. For those who are tired of their denture and want a permanent solution that doesn't involve their teeth coming in and out of their mouth on a daily basis the full mouth hybrid dental bridge is the top of the line Cadillac option. The beauty of this procedure is in most cases it can bypass the terminal dentition patient (one who is losing all remaining teeth due to failing dental work or disease), even going through the low point of having no teeth and complete loss of oral function. What does this mean? It means that they have to go through months of eating through a straw and impaired ability to speak confidently, as well as many other challenges to acclimating to no longer having teeth.

Our solution is made possible through a team effort of a combined dental implant surgeon and dental lab technician teeth in a day outcome. With state of the art imaging and experience, a plan can be made in most cases to give a natural feeling and functioning mouth of teeth that stay in place the same day that the failing teeth are removed. As illustrated in the next images you'll view, the hybrid bridge is held securely in place with special screws and the only way the prosthesis can be removed from the mouth is by the dentist during dental cleaning appointments.

This option is the ultimate upgrade from any type of full mouth denture solution. In addition to being permanently fixed in the mouth this option also allows for far less bulk of material than any denture option, which in turn results in a more natural and comfortable feeling in the mouth. This allows for more natural feeling, chewing, and speech - not to mention much more confidence.

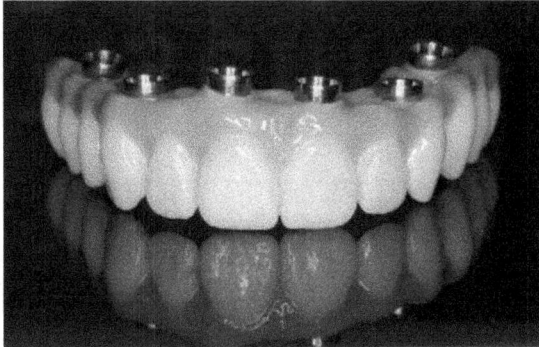

FINDING A QUALIFIED DENTIST

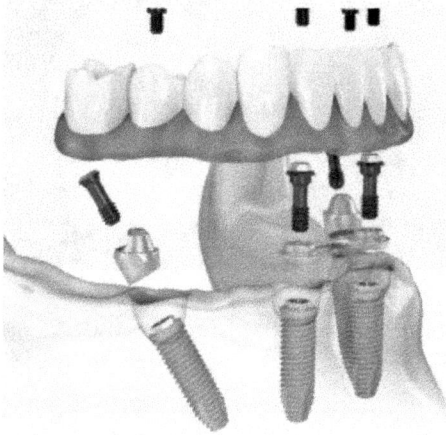

There is no substitute for the right education about dental implants, as it is a precise science and application that takes a great deal of knowledge and understanding about the procedure as a whole, plus the minute details. They all make a difference.

In addition to post-doctoral education, there is also the actual hands-on implant experience. As I'd mentioned earlier, I observed these procedures for years, paying close attention to the best in the industry before I began to offer them. As a result, I was able to start doing dental implants with exceptional results fairly quickly within my practice. The results are so important to me and I'm very appreciative of how all the five star reviews I receive can help to solidify to my patients that they are choosing a professional that not only knows the processes, but that they can trust and will do what they say they'll do.

Another area that you should be very aware of is the technology that a dentist will use in order to ensure they are helping guide you to the best dental implant choices. This involves a very high tech, specific piece of equipment that is called a Cone Beam 3D x-ray machine. The image it provides is detailed and precise, showing the most accurate depiction of what the mouth's condition and challenges are. There is no substitute for it.

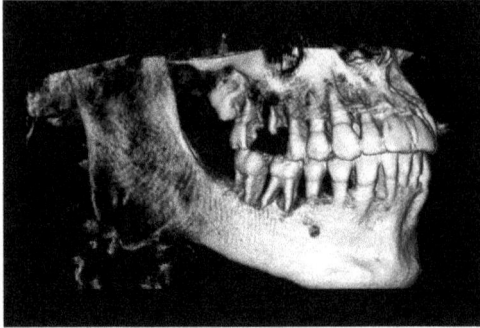

Also, don't hesitate to ask for referrals and do some research, not only on the dentist, but the entire staff. It's a group effort, lead and guided by the dentist, to take care of you. In our office, we treat every consultation and patient with dignity and respect. We are thankful they are there and eager to be of service. It's this type of compassion-based philosophy that has given us the wonderful joy of working with so many different people.

It's also important for you to know that if it is the appropriate move after your consultation and exam, we will refer you to a qualified periodontist or oral surgeon. Sometimes, due to your circumstances, this can be the case and since your wellbeing is our priority, we will make sure we have a complete picture before proceeding. Plus, you must know all your options. Don't settle for anything less from anyone you choose to have a consultation with, should you choose to research multiple places.

PAIN AND DISCOMFORT

You're not alone if you're wondering if it hurts to get dental implants. It's probably the number one question that my staff and I get. Thankfully, we can confidently share with you that it is a less uncomfortable, painful process than you may be imagining. Our experience with implants, combined with our knowledge of sedation dentistry all help to create a tranquil, calming, and pleasant experience for our patients.

The way we manage pain during the procedure is to use local anesthesia to reduce discomfort to a minimum, if at all. When it comes to addressing anxiety, we also have the option to administer nitrous oxide (laughing gas) in conjunction with an anti-anxiety medication, if necessary. If this is done, it often leaves the patient with no memory of the procedure.

After the procedure is complete and the patient is at home healing, most have not required anything other than Advil or Tylenol to feel comfortable. If there are extenuating circumstances, we are very proactive in helping them be addressed.

In addition, we help the healing process go quickly by offering thorough instructions into what will help you most, combined with scheduling follow-up visits with us so we can check on your healing process and answer any additional questions that may surface during your recovery time. We are at your disposal during the critical times too!

Basically...your exciting new beginning should not be a painful one!

Dr. Gates is very friendly and comes in after the hygienist cleans and doesn't just rush in and out, he talks to you and looks over your X-rays. Everyone in the office is super nice and welcoming. So glad my family found him. I can't believe I thought my old dentist gave good service. And now that I've been to Dr. Gates, I can't believe I wasted all that time. Best thing is they do great with pain relief during crowns, root canals, etc. Don't wait if you're thinking about a new dentist or want to change; you won't go wrong with this office.

~ Angela S

CHAPTER 5

WHAT TO EXPECT FROM A DENTAL IMPLANT PROCEDURE

I recently attended an informational seminar at Dr. Gates' office, and I'm so glad I did! On the basis of what I learned there, I decided during a follow-up consultation, to go ahead and have an implant, as well as a tooth crowned. I loved the way he explains everything, and uses the computer screen to illustrate (for us "visual" folks)! At no time was there any pressure from him or his staff. Dr. Gates is so professional and skilled in technique, I was at ease throughout the entire time. He and his assistants were a fine-tuned team, working smoothly and timely at every turn. My initial concerns about nitrous oxide were soon put to rest—and I was relaxed the entire time. A few minutes on pure oxygen (good for humans, I've read) and I was just fine driving myself home. Thought I'd never say this about being in a dental chair, but truly, this was "a great ride"! The whole team is genuinely thoughtful and attentive to patient comfort. Thank you, Dr. Gates.

~ Ruth Galbraith

Your journey to get to the consultation about dental implants has likely been an intensive one. You've probably gone through an array of emotions that include fear, embarrassment, concern, and curiosity. But now, hopefully you've learned enough that you are feeling optimistic about there being a solution that will help you reclaim your smile and improve your health. We're on the same page.

This chapter is all about walking you through the process and what we do to make sure that your decision is one you are comfortable with, as well as one in which you understand the full scope of what you will be going through.

THE EXAMINATION

Through experience and taking into account all the anxieties and anticipations of our patients, the process we go through in order to find out what the best options and solutions are for a patient, and if they are a good candidate for dental implants, all begins with the exam.

The initial exam with a new patient lasts about one hour total. This allows time for us to do a few things:

✓ Learn your history
✓ Hear your concerns
✓ Give you the attention you need

You are not cattle, you're a patient and we value you considering us for your dental needs.

During the exam you will have a comprehensive oral exam, as well as digital x-rays so that we can get the full picture of your current state of oral health. These results are ones that I go over with you, explaining exactly what is happening, and then going through any recommended corrective actions.

If you decide that you'd like to learn more about the specific details of dental implant procedures, those questions will also be answered thoughtfully. We're glad to see you and are appreciative of the time you've booked out for us.

One of the main questions that people have about dental implants is the cost, which can only be addressed after a thorough exam, because it's important to know what specific course of corrective action is suggested. Once that is known, the opportunity to speak with a financial consultant about financing options can take place. With the rise in dental implant procedures, the option for favorable financing from elite implant providers is fantastic. It's a definite perk to working with a top rated, proven provider, which we are so grateful that the Custom Dental of McKinney office is.

FACTORS IN THE FEES

While there is no way to estimate an exact cost without a thorough and comprehensive exam, the specifics that are a part of determining the total cost of dental implants include:

✓ What you need and/or want
✓ The severity of the bone loss
✓ Your choice for replacement teeth

Based on what works for you and all the factors involved in your specific situation, you can determine if dental implants are a feasible route for you to go or if you should begin evaluating other options.

If you have dental insurance you'll have to check and see if any costs of your dental implants would be covered through that. Most plans are designed for preventive care, despite the vast number of benefits of having a dental implant procedure. On the positive side—many flex accounts or HDAs (health distribution account) will allow those funds to go toward dental implants.

You should check out your options that may be available via insurance and your accounts, and we can assist by checking out what options we may be able to offer you, as well.

UNDERSTANDING THE DENTAL IMPLANT PROCESS

Dental implant procedures are a meticulous, tested, and proven process. A great benefit to this is that we can inform our patients of exactly what they can expect if they choose to get the procedure. Because of this, the entire process is a more positive one for you, which is always a part of how we wish to serve you.

In order to alleviate questions, concerns, and the "unknowns," there are several things that you will know before you go into your procedure. They're listed out here and are definitely reinforced throughout your consultations leading up to the procedure day (or days for more intensive work).

✓ With the goal of less anxiety and more excitement in mind, the entire staff of our office is dedicated to creating the most relaxing and calming environment for you.

✓ When it comes to sedation during the procedure, it is highly uncommon for anyone to require more than a local anesthesia.

✓ Before the procedure, you'll learn exactly how to manage your post-procedure care. Taking great care of yourself and following the instructions is a big part of a healthier, less taxing healing process.

✓ You'll know how much time your procedure will take, approximately. On average, it takes about thirty to sixty minutes per implant. Some people choose a more aggressive implant plan if they will require multiple days, and other people move more slowly with their procedures. This is a decision that will be made together.

Through all of this, you also have one of the biggest worries you can have alleviated—you are never without teeth!

RENEWED HOPE AND INSPIRATION

There is a natural process of reflection that takes place as you begin to think about all the lost opportunities you've had in your life because you were embarrassed about your smile or lacked the confidence to allow people to meet the real you—an amazing person that's beautiful on the inside and out!

As you gravitate toward your dental implant solution, you are going to find that you're starting to feel those stirrings of hope once again. Powerful mental images of seeing the people you love most see you for the first time with that wonderful smile upon your face is suddenly exciting. And it should be! If you were to ask anyone if you should do the procedure, everyone would agree that it's a wonderful idea, because you deserve to take care of yourself the way you take such great care of others. To see you smile and be genuinely happy is a fantastic thing.

IT CAN BE AS SIMPLE AS 1, 2, 3, 4, 5

1. Set up an appointment for a consultation.
2. Compile records and x-rays that tell us where you are at that moment in regards to your oral health.
3. Create a customized treatment plan for you, based on your needs.
4. Have the dental implant procedure.
5. Celebrate!

We could have not asked for a better experience! The staff went out of their way to make us feel comfortable. Dr. Gates was very professional and treated us like family. Would highly recommend Custom Dental!
~ Chris C

CHAPTER 6

A NEW BEGINNING AND A CONFIDENT SMILE

This was most definitely the BEST dental experience I have EVER had! Dr. Gates and his team were extremely welcoming and made me feel right at home. During my first orthodontic appointment, I was comfortable and pain free the entire procedure which was something completely new for me. You can tell the team is passionate about giving the highest quality of patient care. Thank you Custom Dental!
~ Brigid Batarse

There is a clear and concise case as to why dental implants are the best solution, whenever possible. Creating a healthier mouth is a sure way to lead a better life. Saying goodbye to the troubles and traumas of missing and failing teeth and hello to a warm, inviting smile that shows people the amazing person you are is a good thing.

Today could be the start of something new for you, something exciting that changes your life for the better—permanently. It costs nothing to make the call and get the information that is pertinent to you, specifically. You will never know what options are out there or how affordable it may be for you to permanently replace your missing or failing teeth with dental implants. No more bone loss. No more muscle atrophy. No more pain when eating certain foods. No more staying in the shadows instead of enjoying the party.

Our smiles are our signatures—something warm and inviting to let people we know understand us better.

It may seem to be selfish to admit it, but your happiness does matter. Nothing brings my staff and I more joy than when we get to see someone, who has already been down the road you're just beginning, smiling at us happily and looking us in the eye. It inspires and touches us, and we're so grateful that we were able to be a part of such a profound solution.

People with dental implants are excited to share how they look, feel, and live better.

Life is constantly changing; why not change your smile to change it for the better? Join the growing number of people who've said, "I wish I'd had done this sooner!"

This trip I had two implants implanted, one would think this would be a very traumatic experience, it is, especially since I am a certified chicken, but I went through the experience without pain and I left the dentist office without pain and slept all night without pain or swelling. The next day I played eighteen holes of golf without discomfort except with my score which is generally the case. I continue to believe this is the best dentist and dental team that I have experienced in my 73 years.

~ James G

About Dr. Bryce Gates

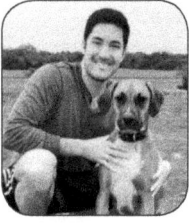

Dr. Bryce Gates brings an extensive amount of expertise and passion for implant dentistry to his Custom Dental practice. Helping people live healthier, more confident lives that bring out their smiles and joy is what inspires him most. By offering the services to do this, he recognizes the importance of providing effective solutions and the latest innovations and technologies to his patients. They deserve nothing less.

Growing up in Carrollton, Texas, Dr. Gates graduated from the top of his class at the University of Central Oklahoma, and then the University of Texas School of Dentistry. Those experiences, combined with his integration into modern dentistry, have led to a commitment to his patients that he demonstrates through participating in extensive post-doctoral studies and industry best practices. This has given him an edge in the evolving dental industry, and particularly in regards to implant dentistry, as well as conscious sedation — a way to take the fear out of the dental work that leads to better health and happiness. That edge, combined with his ability to connect with his patients, makes him one of the most highly referred and rated dentists in the Dallas/ Fort Worth area. To date, Dr. Gates has been involved in placing well over three thousand dental implants.

According to Dr. Gates, "My approach to treating patients' starts by listening to the concerns they are feeling so I can see how to best meet their needs. It's only after this important step that a thorough examination takes place, and then where a serious and thoughtful discussion about the diagnosis and feasible treatment options can occur. Because of this patient first approach, the patients' have a more optimal experience."

When he is not changing lives and changing smiles, Dr. Gates is enthusiastic about the amazing opportunities that are available to him for fun and adventure. He enjoys traveling and exploring with his family, as well as training his dog, Duke. Duke is an officially certified therapy dog and visits local hospitals to bring happiness, relaxation, and smiles to peoples' faces — something that is always inspiring to Dr. Gates.

Dr. Gates also has extensive professional affiliations, including:

✓ American Dental Association (ADA)
✓ Texas Dental Association (TDA)
✓ North Texas Dental Society (NTDS)
✓ Academy of General Dentistry
✓ American Academy of Implant Dentistry (AAID)
✓ The American Orthodontic Society
✓ Frisco Chamber of Commerce

SERVICES AVAILABLE AT CUSTOM DENTAL OF MCKINNEY

Our professional and dedicated team is fully committed to serving our patients and being active participants in our community. Oral health goals are important, as they impact all areas of our life. This includes maintenance dental procedures such as:

- ✓ Teeth cleaning
- ✓ Oral exams
- ✓ Minor dental procedures
- ✓ Pediatric dentistry
- ✓ Sedation dentistry techniques

And extends to:

- ✓ Root canals
- ✓ Caps and crowns
- ✓ Laser gum surgery

Plus, we have the proven, rated experience to help people with more involved dental procedures such as:

- ✓ Cosmetic dentistry
- ✓ Dental implants

✓ Orthodontics
✓ Osseous surgery

Our team will always make you feel welcomed, and you will always be informed. Plus, we stand behind our work, offering a 110% money back guarantee (up to $1,000.00) if you're not completely delighted with your service during your first year.

With our modern, state of the art facility you will instantly feel at ease when you walk in and notice the sense of family—a family that you are a part of. This is what makes the difference for our practice. This is the heart of Custom Dental of McKinney.

Learn more about services available from our dentist in McKinney by scheduling your consultation with Dr. Gates today!

And remember…

Change your smile and you'll change your life.

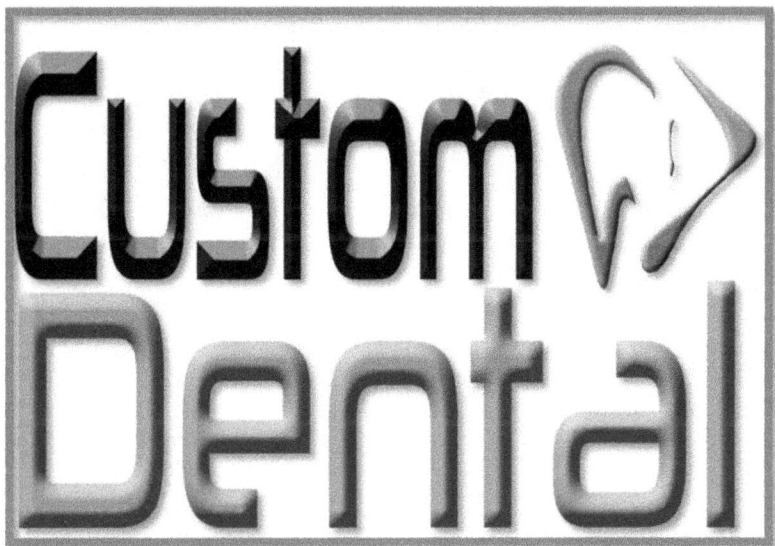

Custom Dental of McKinney
6351 S. Custer Rd. McKinney, TX 75070
New Patients: 469.452.2733
Current Patients: 469.907.1041

www.TheDentistOfMcKinney.com